Alkaline Diet

The Definitive Manual On Nutritious And Effortless
Recipes Promoting Natural Weight Loss And Enhanced
Immunity

I0090369

*(An Assortment Of Thoroughly Explored Plant-Based
Juicing Recipes For Efficient Weight Loss, Detoxification,
And Enhancement Of Overall Well-Being)*

Anthony Beaupre

TABLE OF CONTENT

Cancer Cells Thrive In Environments Characterized By High Acidity And Reduced Oxygen Levels.

In a high oxygen environment, there is an absence of viable cancer cells. Elevated oxygen levels can solely be observed within an alkaline milieu. Cancer cells are characterized by their adaptive capabilities, enabling them to thrive even under tremendously acidic and challenging environmental circumstances. Henceforth, it is imperative that we maintain an alkaline state in order to facilitate a more conducive environment for the flourishing of our robust cells.

A novel perspective on cholesterol" "A fresh approach to understanding cholesterol" "A unique viewpoint on the subject of cholesterol" "A innovative outlook on cholesterol

"The function of blood is:

"In order to facilitate the transportation of the oxygen we respire and the nutrients we metabolize,

To collect the acid waste generated during the energy production process.

To facilitate the transport of waste materials into the body's filtration systems, such as the kidneys.

In relation to this task, the physical structure is enveloped by an intricate system of blood vessels. The blood flows perpetually within this intricate network. In the event of an elevation in the blood's acid load, detrimental effects may arise as the acid begins to inflict damage upon the cellular structure of the vein wall.

We possess the knowledge that acid possesses a positive charge due to the presence of protons, and it displays a propensity for attracting electrons. The acid within the bloodstream seeks out electrons present within the lining of the vein. If this were not ceased, puncturing of the veins would ensue. The human physique serves to obstruct the occurrence of this phenomenon. This is accomplished by occluding the veins with cholesterol. The liver and skeletal system aid in the facilitation of this process. When there is a rise in acid levels within the bloodstream, the liver is stimulated to synthesize an elevated amount of cholesterol. The responsibility of LDL, commonly referred to as the "bad" cholesterol, is to neutralize acid levels within the veins.

The low-density lipoprotein (LDL) that is synthesized as a result of an elevated acid load is transported from the liver to the venous system. It donates electrons to the acid present in the bloodstream. It repairs the endothelial lining of blood vessels that have been corroded due to acidification. Calcium, a crucial alkali mineral, plays a paramount role in assisting LDL in this particular task. Over time, calcium and acid gradually combine, resulting in a solidification process. This leads to the creation of a structure known as 'plaque'. The proliferation of plaque within the veins results in the calcification of vessels, thereby leading to arterial hardening and subsequent complications with blood pressure.

Diagram 4. Arterial calcification resulting from acidification.

Cholesterol plays a crucial role in our overall well-being. It is established that numerous hormones are synthesized from cholesterol, such as oestrogen, testosterone, and progesterone. The liver is responsible for the synthesis of 80% of the body's cholesterol, while the remaining 20% is derived from dietary sources. During the process of acidification, the liver synthesizes additional cholesterol to facilitate the production of low-density lipoproteins (LDL) for transport within the veins. Low-density lipoprotein (LDL) undertakes a self-sacrificial mechanism in order to counteract the acidification process occurring within the veins. The process of acidification of the veins bears resemblance to the process of oxidation.

LDL cholesterol exhibits a comparable structural composition to that of unsaturated fat. All unsaturated fats possess surplus electrons. When electrons are relinquished by them, they undergo oxidation. Low-density lipoprotein operates in a comparable fashion. It undergoes oxidation to prevent the occurrence of veins.

Low-density lipoprotein (LDL) cholesterol transfers its surplus electrons to the acidic components present in the bloodstream, resulting in the neutralization of the acid. Subsequently, in conjunction with calcium, the neutralized acid is deposited as plaques within the walls of the veins. Through this method, the acidity present in the bloodstream is effectively eliminated. Regrettably, this procedure results in the hardening or constriction of blood vessels. These cholesterol plaques pose a significant risk to health.

Through this particular process, the liquid acid present in the bloodstream undergoes a transformation, resulting in the formation of cholesterol plaque, which can be described as solid acids. This serves the dual purpose of averting acidification of blood pH levels as well as preventing puncture of the veins.

Unsaturated fats are recommended for a healthy heart. They provide the same protection against acid damage to veins as LDL does. Nevertheless, saturated fats pose detrimental effects on our physiological well-being.

From a chemical standpoint, the term "saturated" refers to a state wherein the substance is fully occupied by protons. They do not possess any electrons available for donating. Since these fats lack the ability to undergo oxidation on their own, they are incapable of preventing the oxidation of veins, thereby rendering them unable to provide protection for the veins.

To illustrate, fish oil-derived omega 3 is classified as unsaturated and possesses a high electron content. Omega 3 has the ability to accept protons while releasing electrons. Hence, omega 3 possesses the ability to undergo self-oxidation and contribute to the body's protection.

A strong correlation exists between the consumption of appropriate fats and the maintenance of acid-base equilibrium. Saturated fats possess an excess of protons, rendering them acidic, whereas unsaturated fats carry an excess of electrons, conferring an alkaline nature upon them. We will provide a comprehensive discussion of this matter at a later time.

It would seem, therefore, that an underlying factor contributing to elevated levels of cholesterol is poor dietary choices leading to an acidic diet. With an increase in acid load, the liver increases its production of cholesterol. This serves as one of the body's protective measures.

Are cholesterol and LDL truly detrimental to our health?

The phenomenon of vascular disease has been a matter of contention and discussion over an extended period of time. Instead of combatting elevated levels of cholesterol, the resolution to the ongoing discussion could perhaps lie in adopting an alkaline diet to mitigate the acid load responsible for venous acidification.

The consumption of acidifying foods contributes to arterial hardening, rather than foods rich in cholesterol.

Nonetheless, individuals may still develop hardened arteries despite adhering to a diet devoid of fat, abstaining from animal protein consumption (such as red meat and eggs), and solely consuming carbohydrates. This is due to the fact that, as individuals with diabetes are well aware, sugar can also contribute to the hardening of arteries. This matter will be further elaborated upon at a later point.

Osteoporosis

The human body is inherently alkaline in its natural composition. Nonetheless, metabolic processes generate acidic byproducts. On average, the human body generates approximately 70,000 millivolts of protons on a daily basis. This implies that an equivalent quantity of hydrogen ions with a positive charge is generated. The foremost cause of acidification is protons, specifically hydrogen ions. The human body does not retain hydrogen within the bloodstream; instead, it seeks to eliminate it. To achieve this objective, it requires minerals.

Calcium is the dominant mineral within the human body, occupying the highest amount in terms of volume. Calcium is an alkaline substance, and the majority, approximately 99%, is predominantly localized within the skeletal structure.

The remaining calcium is retained within the fluids and tissues of the body. When the pH of the blood and bodily fluids decreases, the calcium present in the bloodstream is utilized to achieve acid-base balance. Nevertheless, should the acidification become more pronounced, depleting the calcium reserves within the bloodstream, the required calcium will be derived at the expense of the teeth and bones, predominantly from the pelvis, long bones, and spinal column. Hence, it is in these particular regions where bone density tests for osteoporosis predominantly exhibit deficiency.

To prevent osteoporosis, it is advised that we consume calcium-rich foods to promote an alkaline state by reducing the acid burden. Through the consumption of calcium-rich food, the body is able to utilize the calcium obtained from these sources rather than depleting calcium reserves stored within the bones. Foods that enhance bone health additionally provide protection against acidification.

Osteoporosis is deemed to be a natural and inevitable consequence of the aging process. Over an extended duration, the human body has resorted to extracting calcium from the skeletal structure as a means to manage elevated levels of acidity, consequently giving rise to the occurrence of osteoporosis. Nonetheless, instead of being unavoidable, osteoporosis can be decelerated and even halted.

Osteoporosis is an unfortunate consequence arising from the long-term consumption of acidic food.

It is a widely acknowledged scientific fact that there exists a significant correlation between osteoporosis and chronic acidification at low levels.

As the severity of osteoporosis increases, there is a corresponding increase in the acid loads present in the body.

Bones serve as reservoirs of alkaline minerals. Magnesium, a vital alkali mineral, is also present in the skeletal structure. In cases of osteoporosis, magnesium and calcium are employed to eliminate the acid burden. The bones account for 80% of the body's magnesium storage. The remaining portion was retained within the muscular tissue. The muscular cramps that manifest in fatigued muscles can be attributed to a lack of magnesium. Fatigued muscles lead to the process of acidification, and magnesium serves to facilitate its neutralization and elimination. 'Restless Leg Syndrome' is likewise an immediate consequence of insufficient magnesium levels. Patients diagnosed with fibromyalgia, as well as those suffering from vascular arteriosclerosis and cardiac valve disorders, also exhibit a deficiency in magnesium.

"Guidelines Pertinent to the Alkaline Diet.

There are certain tips that are specific to the alkaline diet that can help you. Please be mindful of the following points as you embark on this dietary transition:

● Eliminate the consumption of soda and opt for water instead (refer to the infused water recipes provided in chapter six to acquire knowledge on how to prepare them)

• Begin the exploration of sea vegetables as viable substitutes for various food items, such as egg noodles.

• Employ the consumption of gourds and roots to initiate a reduction of carbohydrate intake within your dietary regimen.

• When consuming water, it is advisable to choose water that has been appropriately filtered.

• Limit your consumption of animal proteins to an absolute minimum (at most, one day per week).

• Refrain from alcohol consumption as it exacerbates gastric acidity.

• Begin utilizing spices and herbs to enhance the taste of your food and introduce diversity • Embark on the utilization of spices and herbs to elevate the flavor profile of your dishes and introduce a wider range of flavors •

Commence incorporating spices and herbs into your cooking repertoire to impart flavorful nuances and diversify your culinary creations

● Prior to initiating any supplement regimen, it is imperative that you engage in a discussion with your healthcare provider.

Employ as many of these guidelines as feasible. By implementing these principles from the outset, you will discover that any obstacles encountered can be surmounted with greater ease. Furthermore, it will enable you to maintain unwavering focus towards your objectives. The final suggestion to bear in mind is that in the event of an unintended deviation, refrain from subjecting oneself to undue self-criticism. This happens to everyone. Please promptly rectify your error and resume your adherence to this dietary regimen.

What Is The Relevance Of The Ph Scale And Its Significance In Maintaining Bodily Health?

In more elementary terms, the pH scale denotes the level of acidity or alkalinity exhibited by a substance. To provide further clarity, the pH scale quantifies the presence of hydrogen ions. The pH scale is in the range of 0 to 14, with substances having a pH below 7 being classified as acidic and those above 7 being designated as alkaline.

The pH scale is utilized to gauge the level of acidity or alkalinity of a particular substance. To illustrate this, consider an instance where a substance possesses a pH value of 6.7, which signifies a greater level of acidity compared to another substance presenting a pH value of 6.9.

The pH level of the blood in our body is approximately 7.40, indicating a slightly alkaline nature. When the concentration of acidic compounds rises, the blood acquires a slightly acidic pH. The body attains its innate pH equilibrium through an intricate array of processes. However, it is equally possible to achieve pH regulation through the consumption of nutritious dietary options.

Furthermore, acid and alkalis can be detected in saliva, urine, and various bodily tissues, in addition to blood.

The Consequences of possessing an Acidic Physiological State

Maintaining an appropriate pH balance is the foremost measure in fortifying the body's immunity against illnesses. Microbial organisms such as viruses, bacteria, fungi, and other similar entities prosper under acidic environmental circumstances. Moreover, a higher incidence of cancers has been observed in individuals with alkaline deficiencies. The cellular level of an acidic body is characterized by insufficient levels of oxygen. Inadequate oxygenation compels the body to retain acids within adipose tissue.

Elevated levels of acidity in the body's pH can give rise to adverse consequences such as renal failure, vasoconstriction, and pulmonary collapse. The consumption of various food items can be categorized not only by their food group classification, but also by the specific processing methods they undergo. Certain foods contribute to elevated levels of acidity in the body, whereas others have an alkalizing effect. Nutritional substances undergo metabolic processes and eventually yield residual chemical and metal substances that interact with bodily fluids, resulting in the formation of acidic or alkaline pH levels.

Furthermore, apart from dietary factors, the presence of adverse emotions such as anger, frustration, and anxiety also play a role in creating an acidic internal environment in the body.

Even slight deviations from the standard pH range can result in significant harm to vital organs, including the heart, arteries, muscles, and brain.

Consequences of Imbalanced Body pH Levels

The Significance of Maintaining an Optimal Acid-Alkaline Balance in the Human Body

The maintenance of optimal health relies significantly upon the equilibrium of acid and alkaline levels within the body. Regrettably, numerous individuals endure acid-alkaline imbalances as a result of unfavorable dietary practices and inappropriate food selections.

The human body achieves optimal functioning in an inherent alkaline state. While an excessive alkalinity may also result in illness, the prevailing cause is commonly an excessive acidity, often referred to as acidosis. The consumption of heavily processed, high-fat, high-sugar food, alongside heightened levels of stress, is a contributing factor to the development of acidity.

The consistent presence of acidity due to inadequate dietary practices exerts a direct influence at the cellular level. When observed under a microscope, cells that would typically exhibit robust and clearly delineated structures demonstrate a distorted and irregular appearance.

It is imperative to bear in mind that variations in pH exist among different body parts. Slight alterations in pH levels can significantly impact physiological processes.

The disruption of acid-base equilibrium can lead to a myriad of adverse effects, encompassing:

Cognitive decline arising from delayed neural transmission.

Dental caries, fragile nails and mineral loss.

Exhaustion (your body's capacity for energy production is hindered)

Organ Degeneration and Inflammatory Response - Prolonged acidosis leads to the hardening of organ tissues and the formation of lesions.

Furthermore, the presence of acidic sweat leads to sensations of itchiness, discoloration of the skin, the development of hives, and the onset of eczema. Dysuria (accompanied by a stinging sensation) and compromised immune function are additional potential ramifications of acidosis.

The human body exhibits reduced production of white blood cells and furthermore exhibits diminished immunological prowess in combatting illnesses. Disruptions in acid-alkaline equilibrium yield significant repercussions, impeding the attainment of vitality and overall wellness.

The maintenance of a harmonious equilibrium between acidity and alkalinity is imperative for the attainment of optimal oxygen levels within cellular structures. An environment deprived of oxygen serves as a conducive breeding ground for microorganisms, diseases, and tumors.

Due to the significant impact of pH levels on our overall health and wellness, it is highly recommended to undergo annual pH level testing. One may employ pH strips to ascertain the level of acidity or alkalinity. The alternate choice is known as the 'Venous pH Plasma Test', which necessitates the analysis of blood to obtain precise outcomes.

Adhering to an alkalized diet can effectively counterbalance surplus acidity, leading to heightened immunity against illnesses, optimized enzymatic activity, and an overall state of well-being.

A Comprehensive Analysis of the Acidity/Alkalinity Levels in Various Common Food Items

The initial measure in adhering to an alkalized diet involves the determination of the acidity/alkalinity levels in various food items, particularly those that constitute a substantial portion of our dietary intake. The subsequent delineation of food items based on their acidity-alkalinity will enhance your comprehension of your dietary regimen.

Let us commence our examination by delving deeper into the types of food that have an acid-forming nature. Foods can exhibit acidity as a result of either inherent natural acids or the process of fermentation. Fermentation can be attributed to specific bacteria that generate acid.

Low Acid Foods

List of vegetables: Prepared spinach, kidney beans that have been cooked, string beans, winter squash, corn, lentils that have been boiled, greens such as kale, lettuce and collard. Moreover, asparagus, black beans, and chickpeas.

(Observe the considerable quantity of vegetables present on the low acid catalog?)

Milk and Dairy Products: reduced-fat yogurt, hard-boiled eggs, reduced-fat butter, low-fat cottage cheese, pasteurized milk.

Fruit varieties: Plums, fruit juice concentrate, melons, dates, papayas, currants.

Meat and seafood: Chilled aquatic species such as salmon and cod, as well as venison.

Additional options: Roasted peanuts devoid of moisture, seeds of the sunflower plant, pasta made from whole-wheat, sesame seeds, spreadable fat made from vegetable sources, oil derived from corn, tea leaves, oil extracted from grape seeds, oil obtained from sunflowers, unpolished rice with bran intact, recently harvested dates that are still fresh.

Moderately Acid Foods

Assorted vegetables include peeled potatoes, rhubarb, and a variety of beans such as lima, pinto, and navy beans.

Assorted fruits: Preserved fruit, tart cherries, canned peaches, pineapple, mango, prunes, freshly squeezed fruit juice.

Assortment of nuts and dried fruits: Including cashew nuts, pecans, apricots, and plums.

Poultry and seafood: Turkey, lamb, and chicken

Alternative phrasing in a formal tone: Additional options: Polished rice, refined white sugar and brown sugar, organic oat and rye products, unpasteurized milk, buckwheat groats, wholegrain pasta, wholegrain bread, tomato sauce, creamy salad dressing

Transitioning from a Toxic to a Wholesome Environment

Ought to Be Your Initial Action

It is evident that Steve represents countless individuals, including ourselves, who are endeavoring to regain their well-being. In the context of Diabetes, a definitive correlation between food consumption and overall well-being is readily apparent.

It may not be as readily apparent among the rest of our group.

The central aspect of reducing pH levels necessitates an immediate and comprehensive elimination of specific elements from our dietary intake.

✓ Sugar: It is imperative to significantly reduce the consumption of sugar in your diet. The human body is not naturally adapted for the digestion and assimilation of excessive amounts of sugar, with the ideal limit being a maximum of 2 to 4 teaspoons per day in order to avoid adverse effects on physiological functions.

✓ Enhance alkalinity - similar to Steve, it is recommended to elevate your alkaline levels by consuming a detoxification beverage or kit available at a nearby health food store.

✓ Foods that promote acidity – Gradually reduce and eventually exclude nearly ALL of these food items from your diet over time. Substitute those with foods that are alkaline in nature. We allocate a dedicated chapter to this matter shortly.

✓ Regular physical activity – individuals with high levels of toxins in their bodies can facilitate their own detoxification process by increasing their intake of pure, toxin-free water (ideally filtered through a Berkey water filtration system) and engaging in regular exercise. Commence your fitness journey by engaging in gentle exercises such as introductory yoga poses.

Once you initiate the aforementioned course of action, the subsequent measure is to integrate alkaline foods. Consequently, we have now observed the advantages of adopting the alkaline lifestyle and the simplicity with which it can be embraced by individuals.

Methods to Swiftly Integrate Alkalinity Into Your Daily Routine

We witnessed Steve's remarkable transformation as he transitioned from experiencing disruptive and perilous fluctuations in his blood sugar levels to successfully discontinuing his use of insulin within a span of fewer than 90 days. During this period, there was a transition in his pH levels from acidity to alkalinity, ranging from as low as 6.0 to a normal average of 7.4.

Given that the human body is composed of more than 70% water, it would be advisable for you to introduce potent and all-natural beverages into your daily routine:

➢ Begin by opting for high-quality potable water, then enhance your drinking experience by incorporating slices of lemon, lime, or other extracts derived solely from 100% natural citrus sources into your water, thereby augmenting its flavor profile.

➢ It is advisable to refrain from consuming municipal tap water due to its limited filtration capabilities, as it contains significant amounts of harmful toxins such as industrial runoff, pesticides, and other substances that can detrimentally impact one's health. The topic of fluoride elicits controversy, as numerous assertions have been made regarding its severe detrimental impact on health, encompassing conditions such as diabetes, male infertility, reduced cognitive abilities, and even cancer. On the contrary, when administered in small quantities, fluoride has been demonstrated to significantly enhance dental well-being. The prevailing agreement among experts is that fluoride does not present any significant health risks. Nevertheless, toothpastes that contain the element are mandated by the FDA to display poison warnings. In my viewpoint, fluoride is advantageous when consumed in small quantities, although it is advised not to ingest toothpaste. If you hold apprehension regarding the potential toxicity of fluoride, I recommend acquiring a Berkey filter for purifying your water.

➢ Extensive deliberations were also held concerning the consumption of excessively alkaline water. Given the potential health hazards, it is imperative to carefully consider the substances you are ingesting. You can

Obtain further details from Dr. Mercola's website by visiting the following link: http://articles.mercola.com/sites/articl es/archive/2010/09/11/alkaline-water-interview.aspx

➢ Refrain from consuming artificially flavored beverages and instead opt for water infused with naturally occurring fruits such as apples, avocados, berries, grapes, mango slices, oranges, Playa, pineapple, lime, lemon, pomegranates, and melons, among others.

Essential Alkaline-rich Foods for Integration into Your Dietary Regimen

In the forthcoming section, we will disclose a selection of highly commendable alkaline-rich food items. A great number of these choices exhibit gradients, or are predicated on the magnitude of their alkaline attributes.

Consequently, we shall delve into the realm of foods with high alkaline content, as well as those with a moderate alkaline composition.

Individuals with high intellectual aptitude will utilize both lists in order to enhance nourishment while also ensuring that their body can gradually adapt to the optimal functional pH range of 7.2 to 7.4.

Anticipate initial lower pH readings and remain composed if such results occur. Your dietary pattern will transition from a lower pH balance to elevated levels as you make alterations to your food choices.

Inspirational Insights

If you have firmly resolved to adhere to the Alkaline Diet, it is imperative to bear in mind certain key considerations.

Allow us to begin by inquiring about your shopping inclinations. When you find yourself at the supermarket purchasing fresh produce for your upcoming meal, please remember to exclusively select alkaline products that are certified as completely organic. According to renowned experts worldwide, this factor holds significant importance and must be duly taken into account in the pursuit of an Alkaline diet.

It is imperative to possess a comprehensive understanding of the nature of the soils employed in the cultivation of the vegetables and fruits that one consumes. The alkalinity of the food produced is significantly impacted by the type of soil. This information can readily be obtained through conducting preliminary research on the product in question. Nevertheless, as a customary directive, it is recommended that the ideal pH level for the soil be approximately between 6 and 7, enabling the plant to efficiently assimilate the most favorable nutrient concentrations. In the event that the soil exhibits a pH level below 7, the plant will experience insufficient availability of magnesium and calcium, whereas a pH level above 7 will lead to the plant's deprivation of manganese, iron, zinc, and copper.

Prior to incorporating these recommendations, it may be of value to ascertain your personal pH level. This can be conveniently accomplished by employing a basic pH strip obtainable from any reputable pharmacy. Simply utilize the diagnostic strip by exposing it to your urine or saliva, then proceed to ascertain the matching color between the strip and the accompanying color guide. The optimal time for assessing your pH levels would be the second voided urine sample of the morning. Regarding your saliva, it would be ideal to examine it one hour before having a meal or two hours after finishing a meal. It is recommended that the optimal pH level of your saliva falls within the range of 8.8 to 7.2.

Chapter 1: An Examination of the Alkaline Diet

The human body is inherently designed to uphold a meticulously controlled pH equilibrium through the process of eliminating excessive acidity. The Alkaline diet aims to restore and sustain the appropriate pH level of the body over an extended period. The primary constituents of the Standard American Diet revolve around substances such as refined sugar, white flour, animal-based products, and alcoholic beverages. Our physical systems possess the capability to handle a particular quantity of these food items. Nonetheless, in the event that we consume excessive amounts of acidifying substances and fail to incorporate sufficient quantities of the foods that facilitate our body's capacity to counterbalance acidity, we will experience an imbalance within our bodies.

The human body occasionally encounters difficulty in ridding itself of surplus acid in order to uphold an optimal equilibrium. According to some professionals, it is this lack of equilibrium that is thought to give rise to a multitude of ailments and disorders. The Alkaline diet prioritizes the consumption of foods that contribute to the maintenance of alkaline levels in both the blood and urine. These food items encompass a variety of fruits, vegetables, and specific types of whole grains. This dietary regimen ensures a harmonious equilibrium between acid-forming and alkaline-forming foods, thereby optimizing bodily functions.

What Is pH?

The term pH, derived from "potential of hydrogen," is utilized to gauge the acidic or alkaline nature of a substance, which encompasses the human physique. As the level of acidity in the tissues increases, their registration approaches closer to 0. As the body becomes increasingly alkaline, it registers a greater position on the scale. A value of 7 is deemed to be in a state of neutrality. The pH value is within a range of 0 (indicating complete acidity) to 14 (representing complete alkalinity):

A pH value of 7 indicates a state of neutrality.

An acidic condition is characterized by a pH value below 7.

An alkaline condition is denoted by a pH level exceeding 7.

Certain food items that are part of the Alkaline Diet may possess an acidic pH, such as lemons, yet they impart an alkalizing impact on the body. Therefore, it is not sufficient to solely rely on the pH level of a food to make a decision on its consumption.

The Impact of Food on the Human Body

The eating habits prevalent among individuals in the Western world often lead to an overabundance of acid production once the food has been digested. As a consequence, the urine can potentially attain a slightly excessive acidic nature, thus suggesting an overabundance of acid. It is insufficient to merely kill us; however, it is adequate to engender an imbalance with the potential to precipitate illness. This occurs due to an excessive consumption of foods that possess elevated levels of sugars, fats, and proteins. As these foods are metabolized by your body, acid by-products are generated. The means by which one can render acid neutral is by combining it with a base. Therefore, in order to reduce the acidity load, the human body utilizes alkaline minerals to bind with the surplus acid, allowing for the elimination of said acid from the body. In an individual who is in a state of good health, the physiological processes function to maintain the body within a slightly alkaline spectrum, with a pH level ranging between 7.35 and 7.45. Should your dietary intake exhibit severe imbalance, characterized by an excessive surplus of acidic components and insufficient alkalizing minerals, the physiological capacity to eliminate acid by-products becomes impeded. They accumulate within the cellular structures of your organs and diminish the efficiency and efficacy of physiological processes in your body.

It pertains not solely to the nourishment we consume. Pathogens, environmental contaminants, microbial organisms, and ailments impose an additional burden on our physiological well-being. In response to physical stressors, the body excretes stress hormones, namely adrenaline, cortisol, and insulin. The human body responds by exhibiting a deceleration in the process of digestion. Consequently, there is an extended duration in which the consumed food remains within the stomach, resulting in inadequate digestion. As a result, your body is unable to efficiently derive the essential nutrients from the food required for its recuperation and rejuvenation.

Consuming an excessive amount of acid-producing foods has detrimental effects on your physiological well-being. It is required to exert greater effort in order to uphold equilibrium in pH levels. Engaging in such actions results in the depletion of the body's vital mineral resources and triggers the secretion of stress hormones, which have a significant impact on both the physical and mental well-being. Furthermore, this phenomenon contributes to an increase in body weight and the development of various health complications.

The Alkaline Diet For Optimal Health And Effective Weight Management

There exists a multitude of unconventional dietary approaches in the current market, all claiming to facilitate effective weight loss. Regrettably, an examination of the nutritional composition of certain diets reveals a significant deficiency. If your goal is weight reduction, it is advisable to adopt a nutritionally beneficial dietary regimen, thereby fostering improved overall health rather than solely aiming for a decrease in body weight. The adoption of an alkaline diet offers a beneficial strategy for weight reduction, providing sustained vitality, improved well-being, and enhanced motivation to achieve desired weight loss goals.

Comprehending the Principles of the Alkaline Diet

An alkaline diet sets itself apart from other dietary approaches by placing a primary emphasis on the impact that various foods exert on the acid-alkaline balance within the body. When the process of digestion and metabolism take place in the body, they give rise to what is commonly known as an 'alkaline residue' or 'acidic residue.' The initial pH of the food is not taken into consideration in determining this ultimate impact on the body. Indeed, certain highly acidic food items such as citrus fruits induce an alkalizing effect upon consumption. By consuming a greater proportion of alkaline foods rather than acidic foods, the body's pH can be regulated to reach an optimal level of approximately 7.3. Although this may not be excessively alkaline, it is sufficient to obtain numerous advantageous effects on health.

Utilizing an Alkaline Diet for the Purpose of Weight Loss

Numerous individuals endeavor to follow temporary diet trends or those that pledge swift outcomes in an endeavor to manage their body weight. These dietary plans may yield initial outcomes, yet over the long run, they can contribute to adverse health effects, making them an unhealthy approach to weight loss. Moreover, a substantial number of individuals experience weight regain upon discontinuing their rigorous dietary regimen. When adopting an acid-based diet for the purpose of weight management and control, it entails a shift towards a new way of life. The outcomes may not manifest immediately, however, it is more probable that the weight will not be regained. An alkaline diet consists of foods that are inherently low in calories, predominantly comprising various vegetables and fruits. Numerous food items that possess high levels of fat and calories also exhibit acidifying properties. Consequently, eliminating these particular foods from one's diet will result in a gradual and wholesome reduction in body weight. The aforementioned dietary items encompass red meat, foods rich in fat content, high-fat dairy products like whole milk and cheese, sugar, carbonated beverages, and alcoholic beverages. Upon discontinuing the consumption of these foods, your physiological state shall markedly improve, with decreased acidity levels and consequent weight loss. Due to the nutritional benefits the diet offers, it can be sustained over an extended period of time. Indeed, numerous individuals who embark upon adopting an alkaline diet primarily with the objective of weight loss discover an assortment of additional advantages. Elevated levels of energy, enhanced immunity, and a holistic enhancement in physical health and wellness are some of the myriad advantages one can reap from adhering to an alkaline diet.

Initiating an Alkaline Diet: A Step-by-Step Guide

Numerous individuals observe that commencing an alkaline diet becomes more manageable through the implementation of gradual modifications. Commence by gradually decreasing the quantity of meat, sugar, and fat in your dietary intake, whilst integrating fresh fruits, vegetables, nutritious fats like olive oil, almonds, soy products, and natural alternatives to sugar, such as Stevia. Over the course of time, it is expected that your preferences will evolve, leading you to develop a preference for this particular type of diet.

VII. Ferment Them

Broccoli stalks commonly undergo fermentation to produce pickled varieties. Simply slice the broccoli stems lengthwise and position them inside a jar. Add a sufficient amount of salt to the jar and vigorously shake it in order to ensure proper coating of the stalks.

Please ensure the jar is placed in a refrigerated environment for several hours, after which the accumulated water at the bottom of the jar should be carefully removed. Incorporate garlic, vinegar, and vegetable oil into the mixture and blend thoroughly.

Please ensure that this is refrigerated for several additional hours. Additionally, the fermented broccoli stems are edible.

Maximizing the usage of all components of a vegetable offers benefits both in terms of personal well-being and ecological sustainability.

Incorporating broccoli stems into your meals can prove advantageous in maximizing the nutritional value of your vegetable, optimizing meal cost-efficiency, and curbing waste production at home. This mutually favorable outcome exemplifies a clear win-win situation.

2. New Fruits

Fruits such as apples, plums, pears, and guavas contain gelatin fiber that possesses beneficial properties for cleansing the blood. They not only bind excessive fats in your bloodstream, but also effectively bind and eliminate heavy metals, harmful chemicals, and waste.

Furthermore, the presence of lycopene and glutathione in tomatoes holds considerable value in eliminating toxins and chemicals. Please ensure to incorporate ample quantities of berries such as strawberries, blackberries, and cranberries into your dietary intake, as they greatly contribute to maintaining optimal liver health.

Natural food items such as apples, plums, pears, and guavas contain gelatinous fiber, which is beneficial for blood purification.

3. Green Leafy Vegetables

While you may not possess a particular penchant for green verdant vegetables, it is imperative to convey that these vegetables are abundant in vital nutrients and antioxidants, which effectively ward off the onset of various diseases. Examine the assortment of kale, lettuce, spinach, and mustard greens to ensure optimal circulatory health. These vegetables possess the ability to stimulate hepatic enzymes that facilitate the enhancement of blood detoxification mechanisms.

These green vegetables are known to stimulate the production of compounds in the liver.

4. Beetroot

Beetroot is widely recognized as a notable source of nitrates and antioxidant betalains, which possess the ability to mitigate inflammation and oxidative stress within the liver.

The majority of investigations have suggested that beetroot juice facilitates the augmentation of protein synthesis pertaining to the natural detoxification process of the body. Incorporate beetroots into your salads or pastries.

Beetroot is regarded as a notable source of nitrates and the antioxidant compound betalains.

5.Burdock Root

Guidelines for usage: Burdock root is edible and, when fresh, can be employed in soups, steamed alongside vegetables, and generally encompassed in various culinary preparations.

Dried burdock root is most highly recommended, and its nutritional benefits are maximized when consumed in the form of a tea supplement.

Applications: Furthermore, it is employed in the cleansing of the lymphatic system, detoxification of the liver, hormonal equilibrium, inflammation reduction, enhancement of skin well-being, facilitation of digestion, treatment of gastrointestinal (GI) disorders, and reduction of blood pressure.

6. Dandelion Root

Procedural guidelines for utilization: Brew a beverage using fresh or dehydrated leaves and roots of dandelion.

Applications: In addition, it is employed as a skin astringent, hematinic, for renal and hepatic support, as a digestive aid, for diabetes, hypertension, malignancies, bowel irregularity, and additionally equilibriates the probiotic population in the intestines.

Does this dietary plan align with your personal needs and goals?

Frequently, we encounter individuals offering guidance to each other on achieving good health, maintaining physical fitness, cultivating a slim physique, and embracing wellness as a fundamental guiding principle in life. We also vow to ourselves to adhere to health and diet regimens on the following day. How fervently we prioritize our commitment to wellness! Alas, our faculties succumb to the allure of indulgent cuisine and the contemporary lifestyle. This predisposes us to negative patterns, poor physical well-being, weight increase, stress, and so forth. The allure of slumber compels us to remain in a state of repose, as we opt to indulge in leisure activities such as television viewing and consumption of excess calories, all while promising ourselves a resolute adherence to a strenuous exercise routine on the ensuing day. This creates a detrimental cycle that impacts every aspect of our existence. Inadvertently, we undermine the very basis of our well-being - the intricate ecosystem within ourselves - which possesses the capacity to effortlessly address all of these issues. When developing your 'health regimen', the primary aspect to prioritize is the selection of appropriate dietary choices. That approach offers the most straightforward solution to effectively address the longstanding problems you have been grappling with.

There exists a vast multitude of dietary regimens available. Notwithstanding that reality, a considerable number of individuals consistently fall short of attaining their desired outcomes. However, in contrast to the majority of other dietary regimes, the principles of the Alkaline diet are straightforward: adhere to alkaline foods while refraining from consuming substances that would elevate the acidity levels within your bloodstream.

What significance does the Alkaline diet hold? What factors contribute to its effectiveness? These inquiries pose no difficulty in terms of providing a response. The alkaline diet focuses on attaining weight loss and promoting health by maintaining the pH equilibrium of the blood. To attain your desired weight and sustain good health, it will be necessary for you to address your dietary choices. The alkaline diet regimen enhances the body's capacity to effectively utilize fats, diminishes insulin levels, and curbs the appetite. Initially, it is imperative to comprehend that the process of Alkaline adaptation typically spans a duration of approximately three weeks. You will need to exercise patience. During this time frame, endeavor to achieve equilibrium in your pH levels by minimizing consumption of

61

acidic foods, while incorporating alkaline foods such as fresh fruits and vegetables as substitutes. These food items will effectively promote the restoration of optimal blood pH levels by stimulating cerebral functions. What does it mean? Under typical circumstances, our kidneys are responsible for regulating the levels of electrolytes, including calcium, magnesium, potassium, and sodium. Nevertheless, the consumption of highly acidic foods prompts the utilization of these electrolytes to counteract the inherent acidity.

The Standard American Diet has enacted significant alterations to traditional eating patterns. Pertaining to a nourishing, traditional diet, the ratio of potassium to sodium was historically 10:1. Presently, the aforementioned ratio has diminished to a value of 1:3. The consumption of a diet abundant in sodium, lacking the presence of certain crucial minerals, leads to an escalation in metabolic acidosis. Furthermore, contemporary dietary habits exacerbate the issue by contributing to inadequate nutrient consumption, manifesting in deficiencies of essential elements like potassium and magnesium.

Therefore, the crucial inquiry pertains to the dietary choices that effectively mitigate the acidity within the bloodstream and maintain optimal pH levels. The alkaline diet revolves around the selection of ingested food, emphasizing specific food types. Their significance transcends mere quantification of calories. Therefore, it is imperative to comprehend your dietary requirements. This diet consists of several key elements, namely raw foods, plant-based proteins, fresh fruits and vegetables, detoxifying beverages, and healthful fats.

Raw foods are of utmost significance in the Alkaline diet. Consuming raw and unrefined food items ensures that you obtain essential nutrients, while minimizing the potential hazards associated with ingesting various detrimental additives. Opt for newly harvested alkaline fruits and vegetables, as well as incorporate nuts, seeds, and legumes into your diet. In addition to their pH-balancing properties in the blood, raw foods have been scientifically validated to reduce inflammation, enhance digestion, furnish essential fiber, promote cardiovascular well-being, optimize liver function, shield against various forms of cancer, promote skin clarity, and aid in weight management.

Vegetable-based proteins, such as nuts, seeds, and legumes, inherently possess substantial amounts of protein content, along with a range of other essential nutrients. These food items can be regarded as equivalents when it comes to promoting nourishment and overall well-being. They contain an abundance of phytonutrients that contribute to combating various ailments, as well as dietary fibers that are essential for promoting optimal digestion. Botanicals with high protein content inherently exhibit minimal quantities of cholesterol and sodium, thereby constituting a straightforward regimen for optimal dietary well-being.

Considerable attention and extensive literature have been dedicated to extolling the myriad health advantages associated with the consumption of freshly cultivated fruits and vegetables. Vegetables play a crucial role in maintaining a nutritious dietary intake. They deliver substantial quantities of essential nutrients such as dietary fiber, folate, potassium, magnesium, a diverse range of vitamins, and more. Additionally, a majority of fresh fruits and vegetables offer various essential health advantages that render them undisputed superfoods.

Nutrient-rich smoothies and juices crafted from fresh ingredients provide an optimal choice for a wholesome breakfast or a convenient snack, apt for fostering both physical well-being and a slimmer physique. These highly significant beverages exert a profound influence on one's overall well-being. A single serving of optimally blended detox smoothie possesses the capacity to fulfill a significant portion of your daily requirements for essential vitamins and minerals. With this consideration in mind, I have formulated specialized recipes for Alkaline detox smoothies intended for your consumption. Try them all!

Dietary fats - Lipids possess the capability to combat elevated cholesterol levels, or contribute to their elevation. This outcome is contingent upon the specific types of fats incorporated into one's diet. The term "fat" appears to cause confusion among a majority of individuals, hence my inclination to shed light on a few key aspects. Obesity appears to be a term that instills fear in the majority of individuals. However, one might ponder the underlying reasons behind the significant uproar pertaining to fat.

Initially, it is imperative for you to comprehend this. There exists a discernible disparity between dietary fat and adipose tissue within the human body. Most individuals seem to be frightened by the notion that limited knowledge in the field of nutrition leads them to believe that dietary fat is detrimental to their well-being. This can be regarded as a form of word and image correlation, wherein the word "fat" evokes an automatic association with the fat located on one's abdominal region. Consequently, can a low-fat diet be considered a remedy for various ailments? Prior to providing a response, it is crucial to ascertain whether you are consuming fats that are beneficial for your health.

Despite the negative reputation associated with fats in relation to heart health and obesity, it is worth noting that certain types of fats are necessary for maintaining good health and overall well-being. Dietary fats play a crucial role in facilitating the uptake and utilization of carotenoids as well as fat-soluble vitamins such as vitamins A, D, E, and K.

Provide the body with indispensable fatty acids that it cannot synthesize endogenously, notably omega-3, an unsaturated fat that must be obtained through dietary sources, predominantly found in fish.

Fats possess the capacity to both detrimentally and positively impact our health, contingent upon their fatty acid composition, nutritional worth, and condition. When utilized in its pure, unaltered form, fat provides maximum nutritive advantages. Alternatively, a low-fat diet can potentially undermine our overall well-being and impede weight loss efforts. The alkaline diet supports the consumption of the most healthful types of fats available, namely olive oil, avocado oil, coconut oil, flax oil, grapeseed oil, and hemp oil. All of these are alkaline foods that will contribute to enhancing the nutritional quality of your diet.

With that being stated, it is now appropriate to address the types of foods that should be avoided. Fundamentally, it is imperative to steer clear of substances that tend to elevate the acidity levels within the body. This encompasses refraining from consuming edibles and beverages that possess a pH level of 4.6 or below. This includes:

- All food products that have undergone processing.

- Meat and fish selections, including fresh and processed varieties

- The majority of dairy products - The vast majority of dairy products - A significant proportion of dairy products - A large quantity of dairy products - An abundance of dairy products - A considerable amount of dairy products

Granulated sugar.

- Cereal crops

- All dietary supplements.

- Carbonated beverages and other sweetened drinks

- Beverages with high caffeine content - Stimulant beverages - Drinks containing energizing elements - Refreshments designed to increase mental and physical alertness

Alcoholic beverages" or "Alcohol-containing substances

At this point, you possess a comprehensive grasp of the fundamental principles underlying the Alkaline diet. To an ordinary individual, the concept of 'dieting' typically entails adhering to various commercially prescribed dietary plans like Weight Watchers, Atkins, or South Beach, which may inadvertently expose one to a multitude of additional health concerns. It is necessary to develop an awareness of one's dietary and lifestyle patterns. A nutritious diet does not entail sustenance solely comprised of lettuce or celery sticks! In reality, maintaining a healthy eating regimen requires achieving the appropriate equilibrium by consuming a diverse array of foods that are highly beneficial for the overall functioning of your body, encompassing even some of your personal favorites. This intervention will significantly aid your body in its efforts to achieve improved well-being and weight reduction. It is imperative to comprehend a fundamental aspect – the consumption of food profoundly influences your cellular composition and significantly influences the physiological processes within your organism. Consequently, this factor plays a pivotal role in the onset of weight gain and adverse health conditions. Consume the nourishment that will realign the pH equilibrium of your entire bodily system. By diligently attending to your dietary habits and adopting an appropriate nutrition regimen, you have the potential to significantly enhance your overall health. By adhering to nutritionally balanced dietary patterns, one can sustain optimal levels of health and effectively regulate body weight.

Consuming alkaline foods has been shown to decrease the likelihood of developing various health ailments, including but not limited to heart disease, diabetes, cancer, and a compromised immune system. Moreover, when prepared with suitable recipes, these culinary delights have the potential to delight the whole family.

Can The Alkaline Diet Serve As A Viable Solution?

As previously explained, the alkaline diet aims to maintain a harmonious acid-base balance and substantially decrease persistent hyperacidity.

An alkaline diet fosters an environment wherein detrimental bacteria and fungi are unable to thrive. This leads to a notable enhancement in overall well-being. The adoption of an alkaline diet effectively eliminates an abundance of acidic substances from the body. As reciprocation, the dietary regimen also aims to provide the body with an ample supply of essential minerals, vitamins, and trace elements in order to counterbalance the deficiency resulting from excessive acidification.

Consequently, adhering to an alkaline diet promotes physical fitness, youthfulness, and a slender physique. Indeed, it also serves to deter the onset of chronic ailments and specific indications of the aging process.

Thus far, we have extensively discussed the concept of an alkaline diet. Now, let us delve into more precise details. What are the permissible food choices in an alkaline diet and which ones are advisable to abstain from?

It is equally imperative to maintain a nourishing dietary regimen with an emphasis on alkaline foods. Based on certain online data, it can be deduced that substances such as jam or ice cream possess alkaline properties as well. It is widely understood that consuming such sugary foods contributes to a decreased level of overall health. When discussing alkaline foods, it is necessary for them to exhibit alkalinity across a minimum of eight levels.

To begin with, it is imperative that alkaline foods exhibit a substantial presence of bases, thereby necessitating an abundant supply of alkaline minerals and essential trace elements, such as iron or magnesium.

Furthermore, alkaline foods should possess a limited quantity of amino acids that promote acid formation. The aforementioned amino acids encompass methionine and cysteine, both of which can be sourced from various dietary sources such as meat, fish, eggs, and Brazil nuts.

Furthermore, it is noteworthy that the consumption of alkaline foods significantly contributes to the promotion of alkaline formation within the human body. This implies that food encompasses a compound, such as a bitter compound, that has the capacity to generate alkaline compounds within the human body.

To achieve this objective, alkaline foods should not generate acidic residues during the process of metabolism. These acidic residues are alternatively referred to as slags.

Additionally, alkaline foods possess a multitude of other essential constituents that are beneficial for bodily function. These encompass various elements such as antioxidants, vitamins, secondary plant compounds, as well as other constituents. These substances aid in the process of body detoxification and provide robust support to the immune system. In addition, the body exhibits enhanced capability to neutralize the acids and expel them from the system by means of these various substances. This serves to inhibit and diminish hyperacidity.

An additional benefit associated with alkaline foods lies in their abundant hydration content. The human body receives a significant amount of fluids solely from the consumption of food. Through this mechanism, the kidneys expel acids and waste products from the body with exceptional efficiency.

Furthermore, alkaline foods are rich in beneficial fatty acids, numerous essential nutrients, and potent antioxidants. All of these substances possess properties that are known to exert an anti-inflammatory impact on our physiological systems. Inflammations contribute to the body's acidification, thereby reinforcing the state of chronic hyperacidity. Hence, it is especially beneficial to consume foods that inhibit this phenomenon.

Alimentary well-being can be significantly enhanced by consuming alkaline-rich foods. They contribute to the stabilization of our beneficial intestinal microorganisms, thereby improving the efficiency of acid excretion. Consequently, there is an improved functionality of the digestive system, resulting in reduced production of acids and waste materials.

Tips On The Diet

The effectiveness of the alkaline diet, akin to any other dietary approach, is contingent upon the diligent application of necessary efforts. It is imperative to consider that this diet is an authentic and sustainable dietary approach that should be adhered to indefinitely, rather than a passing trend that can be abandoned after a short period of time. The alkaline diet gained prominent attention in 2013 following Victoria Beckham's endorsement of its beneficial impacts on the physique. Consequently, numerous individuals have embraced this dietary regimen to achieve weight loss and uphold physical fitness.

The diet can be classified as requiring a significant degree of commitment, as individuals must restrict their consumption of various foods that they are accustomed to. This encompasses meat products, drinks containing caffeine, and dairy items. Consequently, it will necessitate additional exertion to embrace the dietary plan and adhere to it. The diet is particularly suited for individuals adhering to a vegetarian or vegan lifestyle as it requires minimal adjustment on their part. However, those who do not follow a vegetarian diet will need to exert effort in order to transition.

You must acquaint yourself with the expenses associated with adopting the dietary plan. You will be delighted to discover that by abstaining from the consumption of meat, dairy, and other acidic foods, you can effectively reduce your expenses on food. However, it will be necessary for you to allocate financial resources towards acquiring alkaline-rich foods in order to ensure that your body receives ample nutrition. Below is a list of actions that you can undertake to adhere to the dietary regimen.

Maintain documentation

A highly effective method for sustaining motivation is to diligently track and document one's ongoing accomplishments and advancements. As you are aware, it is crucial to assess the effectiveness of a dietary plan by periodically monitoring one's weight and other essential parameters. This encompasses the measurement of your weight, as well as the measurements of your waist and hips.

It is also important to periodically assess your cholesterol and blood pressure levels to safeguard your cardiovascular well-being. It is highly recommended that you undergo regular check-ups every few months and maintain a reliable record for the purpose of assessing your progress.

Exercise

Despite not being an inherent component of the dietary regimen, consistent physical activity is essential for the maintenance of an optimal body weight. It is not necessary for you to engage in strenuous physical activities, as you may opt for more gentle forms of exercise. You have the ability to devise a strategy that aligns with the capabilities of your physique. Engaging in a cardiovascular workout, followed by a strength training regimen, will effectively uphold your physical condition. Additionally, incorporating Pilates and yoga into your routine can serve as complementary exercises to enhance your physical well-being.

Purchase high quality, freshly produced items

Acquiring fresh ingredients holds significant importance. The alkaline diet advocates for the consumption of fresh fruits and vegetables due to their elevated nutrient content. Opting for fresh produce on a daily basis is recommended as frozen and dehydrated alternatives may offer insufficient nutritional value for optimal bodily nourishment. One may choose to visit the organic market during the mornings in order to procure fresh produce that can be utilized in culinary pursuits. If you are inclined, you may also cultivate your own alkaline-rich produce, such as carrots, beets, and basil. By employing this method, you will ensure a reliable and uninterrupted provision of these recently harvested vegetables.

Partner up

It would be highly advantageous for you to seek out a companion who can accompany you throughout the duration of the dietary regimen. This individual can assume the role of either a friend, a colleague, or your marital companion.

Both of you may choose to adopt the diet concurrently and serve as sources of mutual encouragement. You may alternate the responsibility of meal preparation to alleviate any potential feelings of burden. You and your partner may also consider hosting social gatherings to impart knowledge about the dietary plan and offer tastefully crafted meals prepared by yourselves to your acquaintances.

Culinary literature

One effective approach to staying committed to the dietary regimen is by engaging in flavor exploration and experimentation. In order to maintain your interest for an extended period, it is imperative that your meal is visually appealing and aesthetically pleasing, characterized by a vibrant and diverse array of colors. Preparing the identical recipes repeatedly can lead to monotony and compromise one's commitment. You are thus required to devise innovative culinary creations that will sustain you for extended periods.

One effective method could be to invest in compelling recipe books. They will furnish you with an ample supply of recipes to sustain you for an extended duration. This book is undoubtedly filled with numerous captivating recipes. However, it is advisable for you to refrain from confining yourself exclusively to these dishes and seek inspiration beyond their boundaries.

Make preparations beforehand.

Engaging in meal prepping in advance will prevent monotony and lethargy. The majority of individuals are culpable of procuring meals from external sources, particularly on days characterized by fatigue. One can avert this by prepping the meals beforehand. One can utilize a slow cooker, which will gradually cook the food. One may incorporate the ingredients into it in the morning and have it prepared by the time they arrive back home. Likewise, you have the option to incorporate the ingredients into it during the evening and have a prepared breakfast by the morning. Additionally, it is permissible for you to transport your meals to your place of work. In this manner, you can avoid the scenario of consuming an overly acidic meal during the midday period.

Profess

It is essential to engage in discussions regarding your dietary choices, their associated advantages, and the advancements you have made. One could create a blog with the purpose of documenting their personal journey and imparting knowledge to others regarding the advantageous aspects of incorporating the said dietary regimen. Additionally, you may utilize your social media platforms to disseminate information regarding your dietary choices to others. This will guarantee a sustained level of interest in the diet for a considerable duration. However, it is important to remain unaffected by any disparaging remarks and develop the ability to disregard them.

Reward

Occasionally, you may choose to indulge in well-deserved treats as a means of acknowledging your commitment to maintaining a healthful dietary regimen. The prize encompasses a range of options based on your preference, such as indulging in a spa retreat or receiving a tangible present. Incentives foster a positive mindset and enhance one's self-assurance. It will contribute to enhanced adherence to the dietary regimen, thus promoting its long-term maintenance.

Here, I present a compilation of activities that can assist you in adhering to the dietary regimen. You have the option to engage in various alternative activities that will assist you in adhering to the diet for an extended period of time.

Lime Green Smoothie

Ingredients

1 cup raw young Thai coconut meat
2 cups baby spinach, firmly packed
1/2 teaspoon probiotic powder
3/4 cup raw coconut water or filtered water
2 cups ice cubes
Pinch of Celtic sea salt
20 drops alcohol-free liquid stevia
2 medium limes, peeled and halved
1 teaspoon lime zest, finely grated
1/2 cucumber, chopped

1 medium avocado, peeled and pitted

Optional

1 tablespoon coconut oil
1/4 cup frozen raw broccoli florets
1 teaspoon wheatgrass powder

Directions

1. Add all the ingredients into a blender and process on high for about 30 to 60 seconds.
2. Once creamy and smooth, add Stevia and then serve.

What Are The Benefits Of Adhering To The Alkaline Diet?

What does it signify to possess alkaline properties?

We aid our bodies in preserving this pH equilibrium through the consumption of a higher proportion of alkaline-producing foods and a reduced intake of acid-producing foods. Aliments with an alkaline-forming effect comprise a wide range of fruits, vegetables, herbs, nuts, seeds, and herbal teas.

Acidic food sources encompass a vast array of grain-based, legume, meat, dairy, fish, fast food, and processed food items.

Ultimately, a physiological state characterized by increased acidity does not align with the principles of a healthy body. Frequently being in an acidic state rather than a neutral one exposes oneself to significantly increased risks of various illnesses, chronic conditions, weight gain, and even prematurely reducing one's lifespan.

Attaining and maintaining optimal bodily function solely relies upon adhering to a proper dietary regimen. An antacid dietary regimen can enhance your energy levels, promote better sleep, decelerate the aging process, safeguard against illness, and maintain cognitive acuity. By adopting a dietary regime primarily consisting of soluble food, accounting for approximately 70-80% of your intake, you can significantly enhance your quality of life.

Significance:
Are you aware that the maintenance of a precise blood pH within a narrow range is imperative to prevent severe illness and mortality? This is an intrinsic aspect of human existence, and our bodies possess a remarkable support mechanism to

maintain the equilibrium of our blood. This apparatus effectively safeguards our circulatory system, albeit occasionally at the expense of our bodily tissues.

When our tissues become acidic, it can subsequently lead to impaired functioning of several major systems, such as organs, digestion, skin integrity, and recovery from injury.

pH is a crucial factor, and there exists a straightforward method to verify your pH levels, along with an uncomplicated approach to rectify it if required.

The internal structure of our body requires a pH level slightly above 7.0. This range is commonly referred to as alkaline. (As an example, mixed-breed dogs maintain an acidic pH range, which is significantly lower on the scale.) Given our human nature, our enzymatic, immunological, and reparative mechanisms all operate most effectively within this critical range.

Nevertheless, our biological processes - encompassing vital functions, tissue regeneration, and food digestion - result in a significant production of acid.

In order to maintain our internal alkaline state, we require a few tools. We are enveloped by a multitude of elements, namely oxygen, water, and minerals with corrosive buffering properties."

Illustrations:

Physical Activity - By engaging in physical movement or practicing physical exercise, our bodies produce lactic acid and carbon dioxide. Lactic acid is inherently acidic, and the carbon dioxide becomes acidic as well, transforming into carbonic acid and water.

Assimilation - The process of breaking down nutrients gives rise to acidic substances. For example, phosphoric acid and sulfuric acid are derived from the decomposition process of the phosphorus and sulfur present in various food sources, such as meats, grains, and beans.

Non-Vulnerable Reactions - The immune system responses, such as allergies and hypersensitivities, directly and indirectly produce significant amounts of acidic byproducts.

Chapter 4: Health Benefits

There exist numerous advantages associated with adhering to a high alkaline diet. One of the most coveted advantages pertains to the capacity to reduce weight without engaging in meticulous calorie tracking and extensive physical activity, thus fostering an enhancement of overall well-being. That being said, it is not to imply that exercise is unnecessary. In order to attain all of the health advantages, it is imperative to integrate a nutritious diet with a physically active and wholesome way of life.

In addition to these mentioned afflictions, it is possible to prevent obesity, known to contribute to the development of diabetes and heart disease, by opting for a nourishing diet abundant in fresh fruits and vegetables. You can avail yourself of this advantage by strictly adhering to the principles of the alkaline diet. Furthermore, it should be emphasized that an excessive presence of acidity within the body has the potential to initiate long-term health complications. Among the indicators that signify the presence of an excessively acidic diet are profound fatigue, dental and periodontal issues, premature aging, discomfort and inflammation, and a proclivity for recurrent illness.

By means of adhering to an alkaline diet, one can potentially rectify excessive acidity within the body, subsequently mitigating the aforementioned health conditions. Take a look at the following aspects that await you once you opt to modify your dietary preferences in accordance with the eating patterns observed by your forebears.

Adhering to an alkaline diet has beneficial effects, particularly in terms of promoting healthier skin with enhanced elasticity, thereby imparting a more youthful appearance. This dietary approach is particularly advantageous for individuals striving to evade premature aging. It should be noted that exposing the cells within your body to an acidic environment can potentially impair their ability to carry out their functions optimally. Due to the diminished capacity of your cells, they will no longer possess the ability to undergo self-repair. One possible way to rephrase this statement in a more formal tone could be: "Consequences arising from this issue would encompass the manifestation of premature indicators associated with aging."

Premature aging is also observed when cells experience inadequate oxygen supply, accompanied by the persistence of toxic substances that have accumulated within the body and its cellular structure over time. All of these situations can be mitigated through adherence to an alkaline diet. It enhances cellular activity, thereby yielding a rejuvenated appearance. Additionally, the advantageous aspect of this dietary regimen lies in its ability to facilitate weight loss, which ultimately contributes to the enhancement of one's physical appearance and youthfulness.

An additional benefit of adhering to an alkaline diet is the enhancement of your immune system, resulting in reduced susceptibility to viral infections. This can be ascribed to the proposition that the dietary regimen operates in upholding the vitality of cells in a wholesome manner. The assimilation of essential nutrients and the excretion of toxins and waste materials can be facilitated by your healthy cells.

Please take note that body cells with reduced strength will not be capable of carrying out their assigned functions effectively. Their lack of proficiency can result in infectious pathogens exacerbating harm to their organisms. An excessively acidic pH level can impair the optimal functioning of your cells. This exacerbates the onset of ailments, infections, and potentially even carcinogenic conditions. To mitigate these potential issues, adhering to an alkaline diet is highly recommended.

You will experience heightened energy levels as an alkaline diet effectively supports optimal cellular functioning, thus significantly enhancing your overall vitality. Please be aware that the presence of unhealthy cells has the potential to impair their capacity to adequately carry and distribute oxygen within the body. The consequences would include a diminished level of vitality and an overwhelming sense of exhaustion.

The cellular production of ATP (adenosine triphosphate), a critical factor in increasing energy levels, is also influenced by the pH level of your body. The production process generally occurs within the cellular mitochondria. The issue arises when there is an acidic pH level, as it hinders the progression of the process.

You will experience a reduced susceptibility to yeast infections – An alkaline diet exhibits a substantial water content, a high concentration of nutrients, and a profusion of essential vitamins, fiber, antioxidants, wholesome fats, and minerals. This feature confers advantages to individuals seeking to avert yeast infections. This particular dietary regimen has the ability to purify your body, devoid of any sugar, and effectively remove harmful toxins and substances from your bloodstream. This facilitates the enhancement of your body's immune system and purifies your digestive system, rendering it impervious to the infiltration of yeast, bacteria, fungi, and mold. The survival of yeast is unattainable in an alkaline and thriving environment.

Your digestion will be facilitated - Complying with an alkaline diet is equally vital in preserving a well-functioning digestive system. Maintaining an alkaline state in the cells of your body can facilitate the process of digestion. The pH level of your body plays a crucial role in regulating your gastrointestinal system. Certain digestive processes, specifically those that take place in the stomach, necessitate a mildly acidic milieu. It is imperative to ensure the prevention of pathogens and germs, as well as the efficient digestion of proteins. Nevertheless, an excessive amount of acidity can impede the functionality of your digestive system. It remains imperative to uphold optimal pH and acidity levels, a goal that can only be achieved through strict adherence to an alkaline diet.

You will experience improved sleep quality - Another advantage of following an alkaline diet is its positive impact on promoting better and higher quality sleep. If you experience difficulty in initiating sleep during the night, it is advisable to investigate whether your present pH or acid-base balance may be contributing to this issue. Please be advised that optimal bodily function is achieved when the tissues maintain a slightly alkaline state. In the event of achieving an optimal acid-alkaline equilibrium within your body, it is probable that you will observe enhancements in your sleep patterns, heightened energy levels, and an overall improvement in your state of well-being.

Body tissues with a mild alkaline condition exhibit oxygen levels that are twenty-fold greater than those found in acidic tissues. Every individual cell exhibits the capacity to proficiently convey and employ energy provided it is situated within an environment that possesses a slightly alkaline nature. An Alkaline body pH can also contribute to improved sleep quality. The primary rationale resides in the interconnectedness of energy levels and the efficacy of sleep. Consuming foods that promote alkalinity can contribute to enhanced energy levels, thereby potentially leading to improved sleep quality.

You have a reduced susceptibility to experiencing symptoms of arthritis – An imbalance in the acid-alkaline level is a significant contributing factor to the onset of arthritis. Arthritis patients also experience pronounced symptoms of the condition as a result of elevated acidity levels in their body. An excess of acidity serves as the primary culprit behind the coexisting inflammation experienced by individuals with arthritis. Alkaline foods have the potential to significantly alleviate the symptoms associated with the condition.

Some of the alkaline foods that are beneficial for individuals with arthritis include green leafy vegetables, wheat grass, barley grass, Aloe Vera, parsley, and alfalfa. In addition, it is imperative for them to ensure an ample intake of water, as it effectively regulates the body's acidity levels.

Mitigate the risk of osteoporosis - Adhering to an alkaline diet can effectively preclude the occurrence of osteoporosis. One explanation for this phenomenon is that the equilibrium of alkalinity in the body is of paramount importance in preserving the integrity and optimal well-being of the skeletal framework. The body's internal milieu must uphold its alkaline equilibrium in order to facilitate optimal functioning. In order for the repair, enzymatic, and immunologic mechanisms within your body to operate at their peak performance, it is imperative for your body to induce an alkaline environment.

An excessive level of acidity within the body gives rise to a myriad of health complications such as decreased muscle mass and bone mineral density, diminished secretion of growth hormone, and the formation of kidney stones. Ensuring the restoration of your body's health-promoting alkaline state through the observance of an alkaline diet is of utmost importance in order to facilitate the regeneration of bone health and prevent the onset of osteoporosis.

You mitigate the possibility of kidney stone formation – By implementing dietary modifications aimed at averting the development of uric acid, amino acid cysteine, and calcium-based mineral build-ups, you can effectively decrease the likelihood of kidney stone occurrence. The consumption of a diet high in acidity has the potential to create an environment conducive to the growth and development of kidney stones.

This outcome can be prevented by adhering to an alkaline diet. Alkaline foods have the potential to effectively inhibit the formation of mineral deposits. This diet plan requires you to avoid or minimize your intake of meat, grains, cheese and poultry to make your urine more alkaline. In addition, it assists in modifying the urinary environment to prevent the recurrence of kidney stones and urinary tract infections.

Enhance oral health by balancing the pH level of your mouth – In the event that your body exhibits an excessively acidic pH level, it is highly likely that the pH level of your mouth would correspondingly be acidic. The issue lies in the fact that an excessive acidity level in the oral cavity facilitates the rapid proliferation of bacteria that contribute to dental and gum issues.

The exponential expansion of these bacteria may instigate a plethora of issues that detrimentally impact your oral health, such as halitosis and periodontal disease. Moreover, this can heighten your susceptibility to dental caries. An encouraging update is that effective measures can now be taken to avert such an occurrence from transpiring in your case. Simply transitioning to a dietary regimen that promotes an alkaline pH level within your body is all that is required. A significant number of individuals have indeed observed pronounced enhancements in their comprehensive oral and dental well-being subsequent to adhering to the program.

These are merely a few of the advantages. You shall experience an improvement in both your physical appearance and overall well-being. When you experience an improvement in your well-being, you are more likely to engage in physical activity, consequently supporting weight loss and promoting good health. You will receive a significant enhancement in self-confidence to correspond to your improved state of physical wellness. Individuals will take note of the enhanced version of yourself, radiating a healthy complexion, and inquire about the actions you have undertaken to bring about such significant changes in your life.

Due to the fact that the alkaline diet can be classified more as a dietary approach than a conventional diet, it lends itself to effortless adherence. You are not abstaining from meals or subjecting yourself to deprivation. You have the capacity to consume an ample amount of nutritious food that will sustain a sense of satiety. There is no need for you to observe with longing as others partake in their meal. It is permissible for you to consume food as well, though it is advised that you exercise prudent judgment in your dietary selections.

Physicians frequently advise individuals undergoing chemotherapy to adopt a diet that is rich in alkaline components. It has been scientifically established that malignant cancer cells thrive on glucose. By eliminating sugar and abstaining from consuming foods that are processed with sugar, the individual undergoing chemotherapy is enhancing the likelihood of therapeutic efficacy.

Osteoporosis.

This publication has served as a preliminary exposition on the measures available for preemptively addressing this condition. It should not serve as a substitute for professional medical advice. In order to receive recommendations that are suitable for your present circumstances, it is advised to always seek the guidance of a qualified healthcare professional.

Guidelines for Alkaline Diet in the Treatment of Osteoporosis.

The optimum dietary approach for the prevention and management of osteoporosis is generally perceived to be an alkaline diet, with a strong focus on the consumption of ample amounts of fruits and vegetables. Regrettably, this particular diet is not widely recognized among the majority of North Americans.

The North American Dietary Pattern

There is an increasing consensus that an optimal diet for individuals with osteoporosis should steer clear of excessive consumption of acid-forming foods and beverages, such as meat, carbonated beverages, and coffee. The National Osteoporosis Foundation cautions in their publication titled "Strategies for Osteoporosis" that excessive intake of protein may have detrimental effects on bone health. Consuming an excessive amount of protein and sodium can lead to increased excretion of calcium through renal processes. Indeed, an individual's daily calcium requirement escalates in direct correlation to the quantity of protein and sodium in their diet."

The Institute of Arthritis and Musculoskeletal and Skin Diseases (NIAMS) restates this cautionary statement: "Although the consumption of a well-rounded diet assists in the absorption of calcium, elevated levels of protein and sodium in the diet are believed to enhance calcium excretion via the renal system." Excessive quantities of these substances should be avoided, particularly in individuals with low calcium intake. The consumption of meat and soda beverages in North America may contribute partially to the elevated prevalence of osteoporosis in comparison to other countries.

Meeting the Recommended Dietary Allowance (RDA) for protein intake entails the consumption of 56 grams per day for men and 46 grams per day for women, sourced from a variety of food options including meat, tofu, eggs, grains, legumes, and dairy products.

According to a report issued by Statistics Canada, the consumption of red meat (which encompasses beef, pork, mutton, and veal) and chicken in Canada has been gradually decreasing since 1999. In 2007, the average consumption per person was approximately 77 pounds (equivalent to 35 kilograms) or an intake of 25 grams of protein daily. (This calculation pertains exclusively to meat and does not take into account other protein-rich foods such as dairy products.) Meat consumption may be experiencing a decline in Canada, however, it is consistently rising in the United States to an exceptional 101 kg (223 pounds) per capita in 2007 - equivalent to 72 grams of protein from meat alone per day, excluding eggs, dairy, grains, or legumes. Given that this encompasses all individuals, regardless of age or gender, it is evident that adults are significantly surpassing the recommended threshold of animal protein consumption.

Beverages such as carbonated soft drinks and coffee

In the field of medical research, a definitive correlation has also been established between the consumption of cola beverages and the development of osteoporosis. It is worth noting that this association pertains specifically to the United States. Nonetheless, the consumption of soft drinks in the country continues to rise, alongside a growing demand for meat products.

A study conducted at the University of North Carolina at Chapel Hill revealed that the consumption of energy derived from soft drinks in the United States witnessed a significant rise of 135 percent during the period spanning approximately from 1977 to 2001. During that period, there was a notable increase in the consumption of soft drinks by young adults aged 19 to 39, which rose from 4.1 percent to 9.8 percent of their total daily calorie intake. The mean daily coffee consumption in the United States, specifically among individuals who consume coffee, is reported to be 3.1 cups, according to the National Coffee Association. Moreover, there is a discernible upward trend in coffee consumption.

As per the information provided by Agriculture and Agri-Food Canada, the per capita consumption of soft drinks in Canada has witnessed a decline over the past decade, albeit remaining at nearly 110 liters per capita in 2006. Soft drinks continue to dominate the beverage market, accounting for the largest market share at 15%. However, there has been a notable rise in the consumption of coffee, which constituted over 14% of the beverage market in 2006. Collectively, these two acid-producing beverages account for nearly 30% of beverages ingested by Canadian individuals. Current research indicates that individuals who are adhering to alkaline diet recommendations for the prevention or treatment of osteoporosis should refrain from consuming cola beverages. Additionally, it is advised that they opt for decaffeinated coffee if they are unable to give up their preference for this beverage. Adopting a more nutritionally balanced approach involves decreasing meat intake in favor of consuming a greater quantity of fruits and vegetables, while also opting for non-caffeinated beverages like green tea.

It is not necessary for us to adopt a vegetarian lifestyle in order to adhere to the alkaline diet recommendations for osteoporosis treatment. However, it is clearly indicated that diminishing our intake of soda and meat while increasing the consumption of vegetables and fruits in our diet is advisable. It is generally recommended to maintain a dietary balance of 20% acid-forming foods (such as grains and protein) and 80% alkaline-forming foods (such as fruits and vegetables). It would be beneficial to incorporate a minimum of two servings of vegetables or fruits into each meal, while limiting daily carbohydrate intake to no more than two servings from sources such as bread, cereal, and pasta.

Opting for alkaline diets is the sole path to adopting a wholesome lifestyle.

The current trends of adhering to low carbohydrate and high protein diets are an invitation to compromised health. All sportsmen and sportswomen are aware that in order to maintain a healthy physique, one must completely avoid such diet plans. Not only do they induce profound exhaustion, but they also prove to be calamitous in terms of weight control. Opting for alkaline diets is the singular approach to attaining both wellness and achieving weight loss.

Alkaline diets necessitate adhering to a lifestyle that is entirely contrary to high protein, low carb diets. The high protein diets induce fatigue and exhaustion in individuals adhering to them. This offering caters to individuals leading a monotonous lifestyle, seeking to reduce their body weight. However, the weight that is shed is promptly regained upon discontinuation of the diet. With alkaline diets, this does not hold true. The diets can be integrated into an individual's lifestyle, and within a short period of time, noticeable improvements become evident. It is necessary to consume approximately 80% alkalizing foods in order to sustain the body's alkaline pH level at 7.4. Diets rich in protein have a tendency to shift the body's pH towards acidity, as opposed to its inherent alkaline inclination. When the body's pH level becomes acidic, it attracts various ailments and diminishes one's energy reserves. The presence of an acidic pH also leads to the rapid deterioration of human body cells. This results in a decreased lifespan. It is advisable to avoid these crash diets and consider pursuing health and vitality through the adoption of alkaline diets.

The consumption of alkaline diets promotes the preservation of the body's alkalinity levels. The different physiological processes are executed seamlessly, while the body's immune system remains robust. In light of these conditions, individuals experience heightened energy as opposed to experiencing fatigue. Furthermore, the weight lost in this manner is effectively maintained and, most importantly, it prevents the occurrence of illnesses in the body. Put simply, they aid in warding off illnesses as opposed to high protein diets, which seem to attract them.

These plans are equally beneficial for individuals enduring chronic ailments such as arthritis, cancer, migraines, sinusitis, and osteoporosis. Adhering to such a disciplined regimen in conjunction with medication aids in combating these diseases at their core.

Alkaline diets primarily consist of a wide variety of fruits and vegetables. It is advisable to ensure a substantial portion of one's dietary intake consists of green vegetables and sweet fruits, accounting for approximately 70 to 80 percent of total food consumption. Lemons and melons are deserving of consumption as well. Almonds, honey, and olive oil are likewise prominent in the hierarchy of foods that should be incorporated into one's dietary regimen when adhering to alkaline diets. Abstaining from the consumption of meat and fats is recommended. All food items that have an acidifying effect, such as coffee, alcohol, meats, and certain vegetables like cooked spinach, should not comprise more than 20% of an individual's dietary intake. Alkaline water is an essential element for individuals who aspire to enhance their dietary habits. Consuming a minimum of 6 to 8 glasses of alkaline water can significantly contribute to the purification of your body. Processed food is notorious for its high acidity and substantial content of weight-promoting substances, thus it is advisable to abstain from its consumption. Beverages such as carbonated sodas possess notably high levels of acidity, and should be completely avoided. One glass of soda can be offset by consuming 32 glasses of water.

Alkaline diets are suitable for individuals of all backgrounds. Every individual should refrain from subjecting their bodies to abuse and instead adopt a lifestyle that prioritizes health and longevity, incorporating alkaline diets as an integral component.

Chapter 4: The Anatomy and Physiology of the Human Gastrointestinal System

The most effective alkaline meal plan incorporates a meticulously balanced diet to promote optimal well-being. Once you have gained a comprehensive understanding of the process of digestion as well as the various roles fulfilled by digestive enzymes, you will be able to strategize the optimal composition of an alkaline meal through the appropriate combination of foods.

The process of digestion initiates in the oral cavity as the food undergoes mixing with saliva, and it progresses through the gastrointestinal tract until expulsion as feces or stool. Enzymes such as amylases or ptyalin facilitate the hydrolysis of complex carbohydrates, transforming them into readily assimilated simple sugars like glucose. Lipases hydrolyze the fats, resulting in the formation of three fatty acids. Peptidases and proteases degrade proteins into constituent amino acids.

The composition of the human digestive system consists of:

Mouth

Throat

Esophagus

Stomach

Small intestine

Large intestine/Colon

Rectum

Anus

The ingestion of food initiates a sequential series of processes within the body, wherein the food interacts with various enzymes at each stage of digestion, resulting in the conversion of nutrients that are readily assimilated by the body for energy utilization, cellular restoration, and growth promotion. Enzymes play a crucial role in facilitating digestion; therefore, the majority of them are secreted within the digestive tract, while some are localized within cells to support cellular viability.

In human beings, the primary site for digestion is situated within the oral cavity, the gastric region, and the confines of the small intestines.

Oral cavity

The process of digestion commences within the oral cavity, wherein a portion of the consumed food undergoes the initial stages of breakdown. When one consumes a meal and engages in the process of mastication, the food is effectively fragmented into a more manageable state, facilitating its subsequent ingestion.

As one masticates the food, it undergoes a process wherein it intertwines with the enzymes contained in saliva, specifically amylase, a secretion synthesized within the salivary glands. Certain types of food undergo complete digestion within the oral cavity. Consequently, when these foods are combined with others that are digested in different parts of the body, a certain degree of confusion can occur, leading to indigestion. This gastric distress results in feelings of discomfort, as well as the onset of various illnesses and diseases.

The process of chewing and the salivary mixing facilitates the food's easy ingestion. It undergoes a transformation into a spherical formation referred to as a bolus, which proceeds through the throat and esophagus for subsequent digestion to occur.

Stomach

The food undergoes mixing and grinding within the gastric cavity. The majority of digestion transpires within the gastric region, thus attributing to the highly acidic pH observed in this physiological compartment. The gastric glands within the stomach secrete potent acid and a variety of enzymes that possess the ability to efficiently digest a wide range of food items. The cells lining the stomach secrete enzymes that facilitate the assimilation of food into the body, promoting growth, repair, and enhanced energy levels. The food undergoes a process of disintegration into a fluid or semi-solid consistency upon entry into the small intestine.

Small intestine

The majority of the process of digestion within the human body occurs in the small intestine. The small intestine comprises of the duodenum, responsible for the digestion of milk, as well as the jejunum and the ileum. The liver discharges bile, whilst the pancreas releases pancreatic juices into the small intestine, with the aim of further breaking down the food to facilitate the absorption and assimilation of nutrients into the bloodstream by the body.

Large intestines

Water and minerals are assimilated by the bloodstream as the ingested food traverses the large intestines. This occurs within the colon.

Anus and Rectum

The excrement or fecal matter, which comprises of bodily waste materials, traverses the rectum and is expelled through the anus.

How To Sustain Optimal Ph Levels

In order to uphold your overall well-being, it is imperative to acquire and sustain the appropriate pH equilibrium within your body. The pH scale is a metric used to ascertain the alkalinity or acidity of a substance. This scale ranges from 0 to 15, wherein lower values indicate acidity and higher values signify alkalinity. Per the information provided on the Natural Health Techniques website by Dr. Deniece Moffat, it is recommended that the optimal pH level for humans falls within the range of 7.3 to 7.6, which is slightly more alkaline.

In the event of excessive acidity in your body, a myriad of health complications can ensue, prompting your body to restore equilibrium by extracting calcium from bones abundant in alkaline substances. That is precisely why individuals who partake in the consumption of acid-producing substances, such as meat and dairy, are inherently more susceptible to developing osteoporosis. As individuals increase their milk consumption, their bodies will consequently extract calcium from their bones in order to restore equilibrium. The Dairy industry, understandably, presents an alternative viewpoint that contradicts the scientifically established facts in order to protect its substantial financial interests.

Step 1

Please obtain a pH kit from a pharmacy that can be utilized on a daily basis. This will provide an indication of the alkalinity level of your body. Alkalinity refers to values on the pH scale that are greater than 7.0. After a period of time, you will develop the ability to perceive and discern the sensations emanating from your physical being.

Step 2

Consume the recommended daily quantity of water on a consistent basis to facilitate the elimination of toxins from your body. According to the guidelines provided by the International Sports Medicine Institute, it is recommended to consume a minimum of 0.5 ounces of water per pound of body weight. Hence, in the event that your weight is 150 pounds, a minimum of 75 ounces of water is required, equivalent to approximately ten glasses with a capacity of eight ounces each.

Step 3

It is recommended that approximately 75 to 85% of our dietary intake consist of high water content foods that possess the ability to generate an alkaline residue in the human body. One can readily obtain the necessary levels of alkalinity (as well as protein) from consuming fruits, legumes, and vegetables.

Step 4

Commence reducing the consumption of foods that produce acidic residues within the body.

Foods with elevated acidity levels consist primarily of dairy products, notably eggs, sour cream, yogurt, and cheese.

Both meat and, indeed, deep water fish. In addition to various grains. Consuming these types of foods in excessive amounts relative to alkaline-rich foods can lead to an increase in the acidity levels within your body. Please be reminded that a ratio of 10 to 1 is required in order to neutralize the effects of acidic foods. To elaborate, let it be known that if an individual were to consume a single acid-producing item, it is imperative that they subsequently consume a minimum of ten alkaline foods in order to maintain proper equilibrium within their bodily system.

Step 5

Exercise daily. Please be mindful that the lymphatic system does not possess a pumping mechanism. In contrast to the circulatory system, which relies on the heart's pumping action to maintain blood flow, the lymphatic system necessitates deep breathing in order to promote circulation and cleansing.

There are no shortcuts. Please make it a routine to engage in moderate physical activity on a daily basis. Engaging in physical activity has the potential to alleviate stress levels, which in turn plays a role in the occurrence of acidic pH levels in the human body. By alleviating stress through the practice of deep breathing for a minimum duration of 20-40 minutes on a daily basis, it is possible to contribute to the augmentation of alkalinity levels within the body.

Attaining the Diet to Maintain Alkaline Balance

There are numerous methods to enhance an individual's well-being. Numerous health professionals contend that an alkaline equilibrium diet is among the methods to achieve this.

The pH scale is utilized to refer to the acidity level within the human body. According to the recorded data, the standard pH level ranges from 7.35 to 7.45, a value that some medical professionals view as exceeding the permissible threshold. The elevated status observed among individuals residing in the Western world can be attributed to the ingestion of edibles with a considerably elevated acidic composition. These comprise of processed foods that possess high levels of saturated fat, alongside dairy products, white rice, coffee, carbonated beverages, sugar, and even fruits like tomatoes and watermelons.

The purpose of an alkaline balance diet is to establish equilibrium in an individual's pH levels. Ideally, an individual whose acid-base balance is proportionate should ideally exhibit a pH reading of approximately 7. In order to attain this level, an individual's dietary regimen ought to encompass a substantial incorporation of nourishing foods, such as lettuce, cucumber, spinach, onion, and broccoli.

Consuming a vegetable salad consisting of these components can be deemed a delectable method of enhancing the alkalinity in one's body. Garlic and mint can be utilized effectively to infuse flavor, while olive oil and citric juices such as lemon or lime, which have a low alkaline content, can be employed excellently as a dressing.

According to certain experts in the field of health, adhering to an alkaline balance diet holds the potential to not only mitigate obesity, but also limit the susceptibility to cancer, cardiovascular ailments, and premature aging. Despite lacking an impact on an individual's pH level, including alkaline-low foods in one's diet consistently promotes good health.

CHAPTER FOUR
The correlation between an alkaline-based dietary approach and the reduction of body weight

What if you were acquainted with a weight management program that would facilitate weight reduction and promote a rejuvenated sensation? Would you try it? The alkaline diet and lifestyle have remained in existence for over six decades, however, a significant number of individuals lack awareness regarding its inherent properties that promote natural, safe, and scientifically supported weight loss.

The alkaline diet should not be dismissed as a marketing ploy or passing trend. It presents a robust and uncomplicated method to experience enhanced levels of wellbeing. In this article, you will gain knowledge on the nature and distinguishing characteristics of this dietary regimen, as well as its potential to yield significant transformative outcomes for your personal well-being, physique, and overall health.

Are you currently experiencing satisfaction with your slender and attractive physique? If that is indeed the case, you are among the minority.

Regrettably, statistics indicate that a staggering proportion of over 65 percent of the American population falls into the categories of either overweight or obese. If one is overweight, they are likely to encounter symptoms of poor health such as fatigue, inflammation, achy joints, and an array of other indicators of suboptimal well-being.

Furthermore, it is conceivable that you may be experiencing a sentiment that suggests relinquishing any hope of attaining the physique that you aspire to and truly deserve. It is possible that you have been informed about your increasing age, yet, that is merely not an accurate statement. Do not believe in that falsehood. Other cultures possess robust elderly individuals who maintain excellent health well into their nineties.

The fact remains that your physical being exhibits remarkable design and any indications of poor well-being serve as clear indicators of an overly acidic state within your bodily chemistry. Your symptoms are indicative of a plea for assistance. This can be attributed to the fact that the human organism does not simply experience sudden breakdowns. Conversely, one's health gradually deteriorates over a period of time until it ultimately succumbs to a state of 'dis-ease'.

What is amiss with the manner in which you are currently partaking in your meals?

The Standard American Diet (S.A.D.) places its emphasis on processed carbohydrates, sugars, alcoholic beverages, meat products, and dairy items. These food items exhibit a high propensity to generate acidity in the body. Conversely, despite the entreaties of nutritional experts, our consumption of alkalizing foods such as fresh fruits, vegetables, nuts, and legumes remains insufficient.

In summary, our S.A.D. lifestyle disrupts the inherent equilibrium of acid-base balance that our bodies necessitate. This condition gives rise to obesity, mild discomfort, recurring illnesses such as colds and flu, and eventually paves the way for the onset of chronic ailments.

We\\\'ve lost our way. This is where an alkaline diet can assist in the restoration of our well-being.

I am confident that you possess knowledge regarding the concept of pH, which denotes the degree of acidity or alkalinity present in something. The measurement of alkalinity is determined on a scale. You have the option to perform a cost-effective and straightforward test in the comfort of your own home to determine the status of your alkalinity level, while also enabling you to regularly keep track of it.

For a minimum duration of 70 years, medical researchers and scientists have been aware of this lesser-known piece of information...it is imperative for your body to maintain a specific pH level, or a delicate equilibrium of its acid-alkaline levels, in order to attain optimal health and vitality.

One may perceive it as unnecessary to acquire knowledge in the field of chemistry. Additionally, how does the appropriate pH balance and alkalinity concern me? These were the inquiries I had initially raised upon learning about the concept of alkaline eating.

We will provide two illustrations highlighting the significance of acidity and alkalinity in the human body.

1. It is commonly understood that the human stomach harbors gastric

acid. In conjunction with enzymes, this acid plays a crucial role in the breakdown of food into fundamental components that can be assimilated by the digestive tract. What would be the implications if our stomachs lacked any acid? We would rapidly succumb to malnutrition since the human body is incapable of efficiently metabolizing a whole portion of meat or any substantial portion of food, for that matter. Does this rationale appear logical?

2: Variations in the acidity or alkalinity levels are necessary for different physiological processes within our body. As an illustration, let us consider the fact that the alkaline level required by your bloodstream is slightly higher compared to the acidity levels of your stomach acids. Suppose your blood had excessive acidity levels? It would essentially erode your veins and arteries, resulting in significant internal bleeding!

While the aforementioned instances serve as evidence that various components or systems in the human body require distinct pH levels, it is unnecessary for us to be concerned about this matter.

Our predicament is straightforward and can be summarized in one sentence - we are consistently exhibiting an excessively acidic state. If you have a desire to gain further knowledge about pH, there is an abundance of information available on the internet by conducting a simple search using the term.

The primary fact that one must be aware of is this. When the pH balance of your body remains acidic for an extended period, it gives rise to numerous health ailments such as obesity, arthritis, decreased bone density, elevated blood pressure, cardiovascular diseases, and stroke. The possibilities are limitless since the body surrenders in its struggle for vitality and enters a state of survival for as long as possible.

Exploration And Comprehension Of The Alkaline Diet

By opting for an alkaline diet, we are essentially consuming the foods that are inherently suitable for our consumption. Upon observation of our ancestors' dietary habits, it becomes apparent that they primarily adhered to an alkaline regimen abundant in fresh produce, including fruits, vegetables, legumes, nuts, and fish. Nevertheless, the prevalent dietary choices of today are replete with detrimental elements such as high levels of unhealthy fats, excessive sodium, cholesterol, and acidifying food items and substances.

The contemporary dietary regimen encompasses a plethora of food items that lack nutritional value and pose risks to one's well-being. The contemporary dietary landscape is distinguished by an excessive consumption of unhealthy food options. As a consequence, there has been a pervasive proliferation of obesity, which has in turn led to a significant upsurge in the prevalence of lifestyle-related ailments like diabetes, coronary diseases, and cancer. The implementation of an alkaline diet can yield extraordinary results in restoring optimal physical well-being, ultimately mitigating the susceptibility to a plethora of diseases.

The alkaline diet is recognized by various alternative titles, including the pH miracle diet, the pH balance diet, or the acid alkaline diet. All the substances that we ingest have an impact on the body's pH balance, either promoting an alkaline or acidic environment. Understanding the concept of an alkaline diet may present challenges for a considerable portion of individuals. The difficulty lies in discerning the foods that possess acidity and those that possess alkalinity.

When the process of digestion and metabolism takes place within the body, it gives rise to what is commonly known as an alkaline residue or acid residue. The initial pH level of the food is not taken into account in the ultimate impact on the body. Indeed, certain highly acidic foods, such as citrus fruits, elicit an alkaline response upon consumption. By consuming a greater proportion of alkaline-rich foods as opposed to acidic foods, it is possible to modulate the body's pH to achieve an optimal level of approximately 7.3. Although this level does not reach a high degree of alkalinity, it is adequate to obtain numerous advantageous effects on one's health.

According to the recommended criteria, an alkaline diet should comprise approximately 75 to 80 percent of foods listed in the alkaline food chart. The primary factor to take into account when embarking on an alkaline diet is to refrain from consuming food substances that are deemed highly acidic. Certain food items are regarded as more acidic or inclined towards acid formation in the body compared to others. Foods with high acidity levels include fried foods, sweeteners, ice cream, beer, soft drinks, table salt, jam, beef, lobster, and processed cheese. Carbonated beverages such as cola exhibit a meticulously determined pH level of 2.5, a level of acidity deemed excessively high.

Contrarily, there exists a category of foods known as alkaline foods. Certain alkaline foods are classified as having high alkalinity, such as sweet potato, sea salt, seaweed, watermelon, pineapple, lime, pumpkin seeds, tangerines, and lentils. As you consume a greater amount of alkaline foods, the body's acidity levels diminish, leading to an enhanced sense of well-being. In an ideal scenario, the pH levels of the body and blood typically fall within the range of 7.35 to 7.45.

There are numerous advantages associated with the alteration of dietary habits from consuming junk food and acidic diets to adopting alkaline diets. The human body, when maintained at its inherent and marginally alkaline condition, is more adept at combatting ailments. When adhering to an alkaline diet, the process of shedding excess weight and effectively managing a healthy body weight is facilitated.

Furthermore, individuals can expect to experience an elevation in their energy levels while simultaneously experiencing a reduction in feelings of anxiety and irritability. There is a reduction in mucous production, leading to nasal congestion relief, when partaking in alkaline diets, consequently facilitating respiration. Allergies may be mitigated by adopting an alkaline dietary regimen. Furthermore, adopting alkaline diets can enhance the body's resilience against ailments such as cancer and diabetes.

The alkaline diet simply requires that we exert a deliberate endeavor to comply with the diet in order to obtain all of these beneficial health outcomes.

Chapter 1: Commencing the Expedition, Fundamentals

Prior to delving into the intricate details of the book, it is imperative for us to convey a significant message to our esteemed readership. Instead of hastily adopting a new dietary regimen and hastily declaring its lack of efficacy after only a brief period, achieving noticeable advancements necessitates unwavering commitment. Short-term benefits can be realized, however, it is crucial to cultivate the motivation to persevere in order to attain enduring outcomes.

Given the proliferation of numerous hot air balloon motivational speakers saturating the market with unproven offerings, it is not surprising that people become increasingly disengaged from motivational speeches. The timeliness of achieving specific goals is contingent upon the manner in which we handle setbacks, whether they are of minimal or significant nature. Having drawn from my extensive expertise, I have synthesized the procedure into the following formula:

The correlation between circumstances and responses is indicative of the resulting outcome.

The manner in which we react to specific circumstances presently unfolding in our lives has a profound impact on the eventual outcome and trajectory of our lives. For instance, the experience of consistently feeling fatigued upon awakening each day suggests that the body is signaling an impending hazard (a situation). To counter this effect, the individual brews a cup of caffeinated drink (apologies to lovers of caffeinated drinks) to reboot the system (response). Engaging in this activity for an extended duration gives rise to health complications.

Nevertheless, opting for an alternative approach in response to the situation of waking up fatigued yields a favorable outcome that ultimately enhances one's overall well-being. One beneficial reaction in this regard pertains to the selection of an improved dietary regimen intended to facilitate nourishment and enhance bodily functions by supplying it with readily combustible fuel, resulting in minimal or negligible residue. Owing to the prevailing conditions of declining health, opting for an alkaline diet yields advantageous results, both in the immediate and the enduring future.

Please bear in mind that our reactions to the circumstances that surround us have a significant impact on the results we achieve, both in the immediate and distant future.